I0435487

I dedicate this book to

my late husband Vinton McClure III

The New Science of Health

By

Slava McClure

Copyright© 2013 Slava McClure. All Rights
Reserved!

Contents

All Matter originates and exists only by virtue of a force. Behind this force is the existence of a conscious and intelligent mind. This mind is the matrix of all matter.

Max Planck

The founder of quantum physics

1. Heart and Brain Coherency

Our body is not made of different parts acting alone, but all the parts in our body work as one system. There is a mind body interaction and this has a lot to do of the development of disease in general.

Stress on the brain will cause output energy into the body, which affects all of our organs.

Some people have the ability to discharge brain stress in various parts of their body and other people channel their stress into usually one area. For example some people get back pain from stress, some people get chest pain from stress, some people get upper neck and headache from stress. This is all channeled energy and distress going to the various parts of the body and manifesting as physical findings and signs from stress, being channeled and discharged elsewhere, because the brain has only certain capacity to hold on to that energy and then it has to discharge it into the body.

As you see there is a definite mind body interaction. Many people channel their stress into the heart and scientists know that the stress and adrenalin that is being produced by stress goes into the heart and affects it in an adverse way that can create abnormal heart rhythms, spasms of the arteries of the heart and even clogging up the arteries of the heart. The heart is an electrical organ. It produces bio-electricity in our body up to 40 times stronger than the brain. This electrical energy travels in every single cell in our body. It is strong enough that can be detected outside of our body beyond the skin. The heart produces electromagnetic field that surrounds our body in 360 degrees and it can be detected about 3 feet outside of our body.

The human nervous system is an electrical system where positive and negative ions flow. The frequencies of the field of the heart change depending upon what we are feeling. Our emotional state influences changes into that electro-magnetic field. For instance if we are feeling strong negative emotion like anger, this creates an incoherent spectrum in that field and many different frequencies start to fight for power. When we are feeling positive emotions like appreciation or love, that electro-magnetic field creates a harmonic spectrum, because the frequencies are working together in a harmonic sequence. If we take that a step further, what we do is we are broadcasting this energy into our body, and we are also sending it out into the space.

2. Excess weight

As I mentioned earlier our body organs work as one system. For example without a proper level of power, the liver will be weak to perform its functions, and without the proper message the organ itself will not know what to do. This can cause to the body excess weight. Healthy body does not suffer from excess weight. Excess weight is considered as a symptom of a health issue and the problem lies inside your body. Excess weight is an external symptom of a deeper imbalance between different organs such as the spleen and the liver. Other reason for excess weight could be eating too many dairy products which cause mucus problem, which on the other hand causes disfunction of the spleen or the lungs. If so unless you restore the relationship between these two organs it is unlikely that you will be able to take off the weight you want or keep it off.

Your body should be able to process smoothly and eventually let go of everything that enters it – not only food, but emotions as well, because the food itself is not the only problem.

3. DNA

As you can see we move far beyond our biology into the quantum physics to understand how the fields that we produce with our thoughts and emotions affect our health.

As human beings each one of us is characterized by his own frequencies, which are the mirror of the proteins created into our bodies.

Our DNA represents our entire genetic blue print. It is here that everything about us is represented as information in a DNA matrix code language. Our destiny appears fixed because of this blue print.

Dr. Frits Albert Popp has discovered the bio-photons in 1976 and proved the existing of human light emissions emitted from our DNA, the co-reactor from where we are broadcasting our unique energy signature.

Dr. Bruce Lipton has made a revolutionary discovery and first proved that the DNA nucleus is not the brain of the cell, but rather the intelligent center of the cell is the membrane. The membrane receives signals from our consciousness and writes the DNA code. For the first time in history Dr. Bruce Lipton proved that we can actually re-program our DNA if we are dissatisfied with our blueprint and broadcast a new message about ourselves into the Universe, because the membrane of the human cell is an information processor and it acts like a semi-conductor with gates and channels. The cell is an information processor because the membrane reads the environment and adjusts our biology. The nucleus of the cell with its gens can read and write, so basically the cell is a programmable device. We can put it into an environment and it will read it, and then adjust the expression of the gens to match the needs of that environment.

Taking genetic cells and putting one cell into a culture with certain environmental conditions causes the cell to program itself (for example as a muscle cell), and a genetically identical cell put into another environment by reading it to express a bone cell. What we are saying is that basically the cells are reprogrammable and respond to environmental information.

If we put a culture dish of cells into an adverse environment, than what would have happen is these cells will get sick, and eventually die, and if we move that very same culture dish into a healthy environment the same cells would immediately recover and the culture will flourish. The relevance about all this is that we go back of the nature of the human being and recognize that, containing 50 trillion cells, the human body is a skin covered dish.

If you put your body into the same adverse environment the body will get sick, and if you put it into a healthy environment, it will recover itself and begin to flourish again.

Each cell has many proteins inside and each protein has its own structure and function. The proteins have different shape and polarity, because they are made of 20 different amino-acids and each amino-acid has its own shape.

Every signal coming from the environment bounces to a protein and changes the charge of the back bone of the protein, and makes the protein to move and to change its shape. This movement tells the cell to do its work (respiration, digestion, etc.). When the signal stops, also stops the movement of the protein. If we want to see another movement, we put another signal. In other words we can control the behavior of the proteins.

The DNA is only the blueprint of our body.

When we open the nucleus of a cell, we will see there 23 pairs of chromosomes (23 from your mother and 23 from your father). Our chromosomes are made of 50 percent DNA and 50 percent proteins. If one of the proteins is missing and we need to make another one, that is when we need the DNA. This 50 percent of the protein is not just space filler. The new studies have discovered that proteins form a sleeve around the DNA, so when we want to read the gen we have to remove the sleeve of the proteins first. This new science is called Epigenetic Control. Epi means above, so literally the word epigenetic means control above the gens. When a signal comes from the field it bumps into a regulatory protein and changes the shape of the protein. When the shape changes, the sleeve pops off and then we can read the gens. At that moment when the gens can be red another protein comes and makes a copy of the gen. This copy is called RNA and goes into the cells, used as a blueprint. As you see the gens have no control over our health and behavior. These are over thirty thousand different proteins in a gen.

As we can see our state of health is a reflection of the environment that we live in, and the environment that we perceive.

If we can summarize this we must say that our believes have a profound impact on our body chemistry.

Self-believe is closely linked to the neuro-transmitter serotonin, and the lack of it can cause severe proportions, and it can lead to depression and self-destructive behaviors. The Universal truth is that everything is energy and we live in an illusion that everything is matter, but the truth is that if you look at the quantum atom it has no structure. Every atom is a spinning field and creates waves and their waves interact. These waves are called the field. So matter and filed equals structure. Albert Einstein said that the field is the soul governing agency of the particle or matter.

4. The Brain

Each neuron produces a charge measured in voltage which can change when ions flow in and out of the cell. Once a neuron's voltage reaches a certain level it will fire an electrical signal to other cells, which will repeat the process. When many neurons fire at the same time we can measure these changes in a form of a wave. Brain waves underpin everything that is going on in our mind. As the neurons oscillate different frequencies, they get classified in bands as alpha, theta and gamma. Each of them is associated with different tasks. Brain waves allow brain cells to tune into the frequency corresponding to their particular task.

We are a global network of neuro-chemical reactions. When we change the field, we change the atom and the physical reality around us, so we can heal our bodies, because our physical body is the mirror of something that is not so physical.

5. The Mind

The mind is controlling our biology. In later years you have probably heard of stem cells.

What is a stem cell?

Your body is completely covered in stem cells. They can replace any tissue or organ in your body. We use to think that the heart can't regenerate, but now we know that this is possible. Stem cells are found in every tissue and organ, but the strange thing is they do not work for us. Why? The answer is because of genetic and believes. For example if you believe that you can't heal yourself, this is what stopped the action of the stem cells.

We have talked about how the signals make the protein to move. These signals are created by the field. The signals can be caused by three things: trauma, toxins, which cause us the disease. The thoughts are the most important thing we are talking about in this chapter because the mind is the governing device of life.

The conclusion is that the gens do not control our behavior. We are controlled by our perception of the environment or in other words, we are not limited by our gens, but we are limited by our perception.

That's why it is so wrong to think that if your parents have certain disease you are going to get it too. This is what we were forced to believe up until now. For example when we talk about cancer the simple truth is this: less that 10 percent of cancer has a hereditary basis to it, and 90 percent of the cancer is related to the environmental lifestyle. It is important for you to understand this clearly – the cancer gen does not mean you have cancer, it is simply means you have previous position of cancer.

The thought is the image of the quantum possibility. In other words there are many possibilities and we have to reach end of these possibilities with our mind. We have to lock in only one of the possibilities. This means we have taken it and identified it so we can bring this quantum possibility into a quantum reality in our everyday lives. This is why our self a steam is so important – you create the feeling trough your thoughts, which leads to the results you want. If the thoughts have no feeling, they are called an empty affirmation. Your thoughts and emotions create the feeling and as the three become one, that you can start to manifest the healing and the things you desire. This is not something that you do for a minute and then you just walk away, rather is something that you become, as if these experiences you want are already happening in your life and they happen very quickly for some people. It is all about clarity and specificity. The feelings are the union of the thoughts and the emotions. Scientifically it appears that this field or this mirror, created from the mind, the emotions and the feelings, is a mirror and a bridge between our inner and our outer world. It can give as only what we give it to work with.

This is the great secret that was edited out of our Christian and Pre-Christian traditions.

What we are beginning to understand is that our human emotions are the language that our field recognizes and the field works in what we call real time. The field does not know 30 minutes from now, so if you say for example I want to be healthy in about 30 minutes from now, it does not know "the 30 minutes from now". This is a real time application!

6. The Emotions

The emotions are a language and the power of human emotions, that we typically discount, can change the reality we live in, or the conditions of the healing in our body. This power has the ability to influence not only our bodies biologically, but beyond our bodies into the physical world on a quantum level.

Too many people discount the effect of the things that can't be seen. The power of human emotions is among these things that cannot be seen.

The facts now show that the human emotions change our DNA and the way our body functions and those effects extend beyond our body into the physical matter.

Our body stores energy, but it also releases energy. Every cell in our body has about 1.17 V of electrical potential, but we have about fifty trillion cells, so doing the math fifty trillion times 1.17 equals tremendous amount of potential power.

The researchers now show us that we can change either the magnetic field of an atom, or the electrical field of the atom and by doing so, we literally change that atom, as a response of the emotions that we create. This is a field of energy that underlies all physical reality and only now we are beginning to understand it how it works. We now understand that the feelings are creating a pattern of magnetic and electrical field of our heart, allowing the pattern to appear as a physical manifestation.

7. The Food

Hippocrates believed that the human body has an infinite capacity of healing itself. We cannot talk about self-healing and not to talk about nutrition.

Today heart disease and cancer are the top two killers in the world.

When it comes to your health food does matter. You should ask yourself how much nutrition value you get from your food, because as we talked earlier in the book, the food is a part of the environment, which your body is constantly scanning and directing messages to your body.

Most of the food you find in stores has been processed and therefore most of the nutrition in this food simply disappears by the time you serve it on your table. Most of the fruits and vegetables have been strayed with all kinds of pesticides, but one of the major problems is the soil and what they do to it, because the soil is used and used and the nutrition was taken out of the soil.

We do need to know what we are eating. The so called fertilizer is made of Nitrogen, Phosphorus and Potassium basically, but the soil requires many more minerals. The result of the missing minerals is that when the soil is deficient, the plants are also deficient and then the plants are getting sick or die.

So even if we eat only vegetarian commercial food, what we actually eat is a toxic food.

When you cook your food you lose the enzymes in it. The enzymes are the workers who help your body with the digestion and the use of the nutrition in the food, therefore raw food should be a big part of your every day diet. When you cook your food your immune system sees it as a toxin, because the food structure is destroyed in a way, that your body cannot recognize it. It has been discovered that if you cook more than 50 percent of your food, then your body will not get the nutrition it needs. What this means is that if you eat more than 50 percent raw food, your white blood cells will not get into a reaction to defend your body. This fact led people to discover that certain foods have more minerals and vitamins than others, such as raw honey for example. Raw vegetables and fruits are the key to your perfect health, because we can get all the proteins we need from these sources. They are completely absorbable. For example a steak requires a massive amount of energy to get liquefied in your body to make it absorbable by your digestive system.

Cacao beans are full of mineral content such as Magnesium, Zink, Copper, Vitamin C, etc. All processed chocolate has no vitamin C though, because the molecule of vitamin C is very unstable and once you cook the chocolate it gets destroyed. Cacao beans also have anti-oxygen content that protects our DNA. Vitamin C is anti-toxin, anti-histamine, regulates blood sugar, helps to evaluate mood for people who are depressed.

Vitamin E is good for heart disease, for healing burns, reduces the signs of epilepsy.

Most people do not know how important vitamins are, they can prevent illnesses and they can also treat illnesses. The reason one vitamin can cure so many illnesses is because the deficiency of one vitamin in your body can cause many illnesses. These are only about twenty-four nutrients, but in your body there are many chemical reactions, so one vitamin is involved in multiple reactions. It is the same with the minerals.

Your body cannot heal itself selectively. For example many people have multiple diseases such as diabetes, high blood pressure, and other pains and so on. When your body heals itself, it heals everything and all the problems disappear. It can't heal one disease and keep the others.

You nourish your body with feelings and the food you eat, and your body fixes itself. When people take vitamins, the vitamins themselves do not heal you, but they enable your immune system to do it.

Your body has its own healing mechanism regarding of what you call the disease.

If you produce a lot of adrenalin because of stress, you will be breaking the vitamin C molecule, and this would be the cause of a heart attack for example. You should know that cardio-vascular disease is reversible by putting the patient on a strict vegetarian diet, loading it with vitamins and minerals. These people are able to heal themselves in about a year, without the need of a surgery. Did I mention it is safer? Did I mention it is cheaper? And it works very well. What would happen if everybody eats fresh organic food is, we will have an epidemic of health.

I should mention that when you stop putting toxins into your body, they start to come out, so if you change your diet to eat all organic food, you will be releasing these poisons. We have to get the toxins out in order to allow the nutrition to get into the tissue. The simplest way to get rid of toxins is to drink water before you have your food.

The human body has so powerful defenses for example, that healthy body cannot and will not develop cancer or any chronic diseases for that matter, not only that, but with a good organic diet you it can reverse these diseases.

As we talked earlier your body is made of about fifty trillion cells and the fate of those cells is controlled by the blood. The cell responds to the culture medium, which is your blood. On the other hand the blood is controlled by the nutrition, but there are also environmental signals to tell your cell how to respond to the environment.

8. The Field

People who are terminally ill and become healthy, how do they do that? They change their field trough their mind and feelings, and from there, they change their DNA by chemical reactions in their body. The signals simply control the behavior and the genetic activity. You are programming your cells without even knowing it, because you create a culture environment that nourishes itself by Dopamine, Growth Hormone, etc.

In stress you release stress hormones which cause the cell to become ill.

Basically your mind creates a coherent pattern between your feelings and the environment and then sends the chemistry to your cells.

Each moment that we live is mirrored to us, this is our reflected reality by our thoughts, feelings and actions we take, so what we see is a mirror of what we are at that very moment and the people you are surrounded with mirror our vibrations. This is called a reflected reality.

What is the environment? It is the food we eat, the world we live in, the pollution in the air, the water pollution, and the relationships with other people, but the most important environment is the one we perceive. This is the source that controls the genetics. Think of it, our liver for example can't read the environment, but it can sense it trough our nervous system. Our nervous system reads the environment and then passes along the information to the cells. The mind interprets the signals. If you put stress into your system, it changes the biology and the immune system. In fact the stress is the primary issue of almost all of the disease today, because it directly results a shutting down of your immune system.

Take care of your environment and your thinking and your cells will respond immediately.

During 1930s there were two ways of treating cancer – radiation and chemotherapy. Guess what, today the picture has not changed.

Through the eyes of the quantum physics the energy is the thing that shapes matter, and that is why the energy is so important.

We all have experiences in our lives which are continuously affecting our physical world, whether we are conscious of it or not, therefore I have decided to introduce you here in my book with the ancient philosophy called feng shui which also studies the field around us and affects us every single day.

9. The Compass

The whole system of feng shui is based on very accurate mathematic calculations. All of them rely on the compass bearing. The compass itself is a very precise instrument, which shows you the eight major directions. Each one of them takes exactly 45 degrees of the compass and it is further more separated on three sub-directions, 15 degrees each. Here is an example: North (337.5 degrees – 22.5 degrees) is further divided to: North 1 (337.5 degrees -352.5 degrees); North 2 (352.5 degrees – 7.5 degrees); North 3 (7.5 degrees - 22.5 degrees). On the image below you can see the bearing between each one of the eight major directions.

SE		S		SW
	112.5-157.5	157.5-202.5	202.5-247.5	
E				
	67.5-112.5		247.5-292.5	
	22.5-67.5	337.5-22.5	292.5-337.5	
NE		N		NW

If you take north for example its bearing is between 337.5-22.5 of the compass. 337.5 are divided to:

$$337.5=3+3+7+5=18=1+8=9$$

$$22.5=2+2+5=9$$

You can divide all of the other directions in the same way and the end result will always equal 9, because all the directions of the compass are mathematically equally balanced.

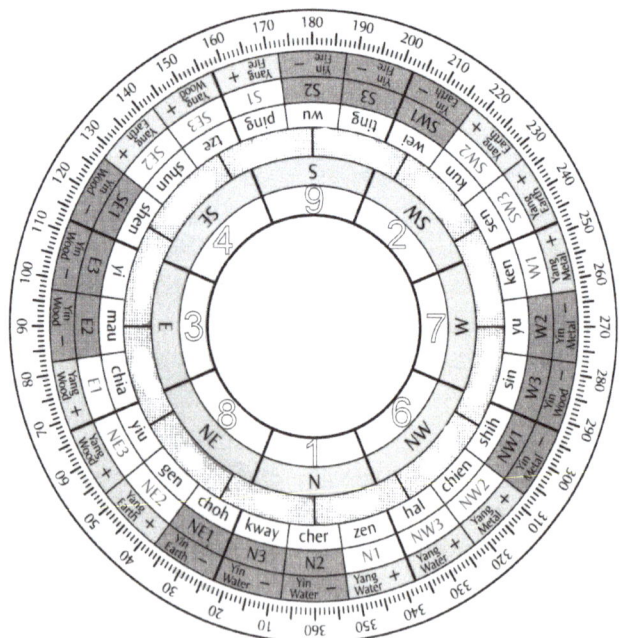

10. The vibrations of the trigrams

Based on the images you saw above and observation on how everything works in the Universe the ancient Chinese people have created trigrams, each one representing symbolically different vibration of a certain compass direction, and they have arranged them in so called Early Heaven Arrangement and Later Heaven Arrangement, both of which are the base of all the formulas in feng shui.

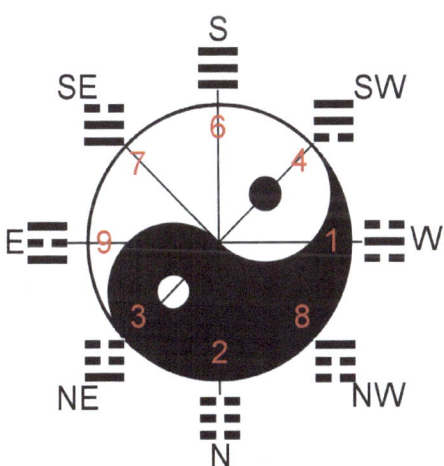

Early Heaven Arrangement

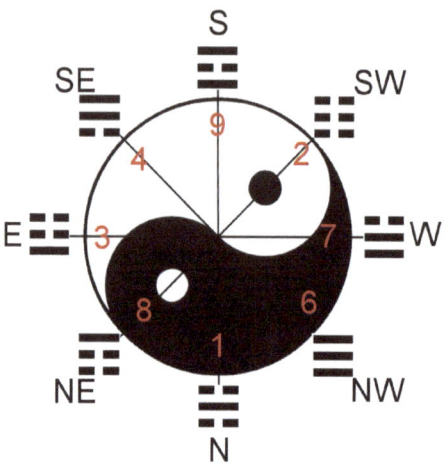

Later Heaven Arrangement

The Early Heaven Arrangement is the image of Yin / Yang – the two opposites, the polarities which are completely balanced. This theory is based on the polarity of things. Everything in the Universe has its opposite like day and night, male and female, etc. The ancient Chinese using the Early Heaven Arrangement and the compass have created the Later Heaven Arrangement concentrating in the center the number 5, arranging them as follows:

5+4=9 clockwise

5+2=7 clockwise

5+3=8 counterclockwise

5+1=6 counterclockwise

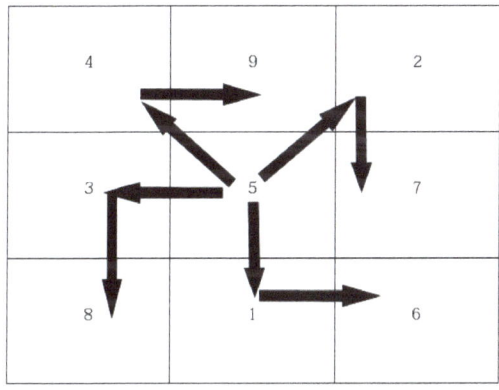

Of course each one of these numbers represents a trigram and you have to become very familiar with their meanings before you dive deeply into the ocean of the formulas here. All of the trigrams are made of broken and unbroken likes. The broken likes represent Yin (the material), and the unbroken lines represent Yang (the potential energy), the ether.

1 Kan	The trigram Kan affects mostly the middle son of the family and represents hard work. Its color is red in the interior.
2 Kun	The trigram Kun affects the mother of the family, the female, the fertility. Its color is yellow.
3 Chen	The trigram Chen affects the oldest son in the household. Its color is dark yellow.
4 Sun	The trigram Sun affects the eldest daughter of the family and its color is white.

5	Number 5 has no trigram, but in feng shui is associated with the trigram Kun (2).
6 Chien	The trigram Chien affects the father of the family and its color is white.
7 Tui	The trigram Tui affects the youngest daughter of the household. Its color is white.
8 Ken	The trigram ken affects the youngest son of the family. Its color is yellow.
9 Li	The trigram Li represents the middle daughter of the household. Its color is white.

Later on I will show you how these trigrams interact with each other inside your home and more important, how to take advantage of them and enjoy lots of benefits in your life.

In order to know what type of vibrations you have inside your space, you need to know a few things in advance:

1. Supply yourself with a accurate compass;
2. You will have to find out what is the Period of the building;
3. You have to find the facing direction of the whole building.
4. You have to mark the sections in the building and spread the trigrams in each sector.
5. You have to activate or exhaust each one of the sectors depending on whether you want to enjoy the benefits from the good vibrations or exhaust the vibrations if they have the potential energy to harm you.

11. What is a Period of a building

What is a Period of a building and how do you find it?

In the Universe there are cycles. In feng shui there are cycles too, each one with the continuation of nineteen years. You will ask why exactly 19 years and the answer is because the basic time cycles are found in the Sun and the Moon. The Solar cycle (year - 365 days) and the Lunar cycle (year – 354 days) combine to form a larger cycle of nineteen years. This cycle is called a Metonic cycle. After the 19th year of the Metonic cycle the full moon appears on the same day of the year as on the beginning of the cycle. In the same way the Sun and the Moon combine symbolically to form a hexagram (two trigrams) of 6 unbroken lines.

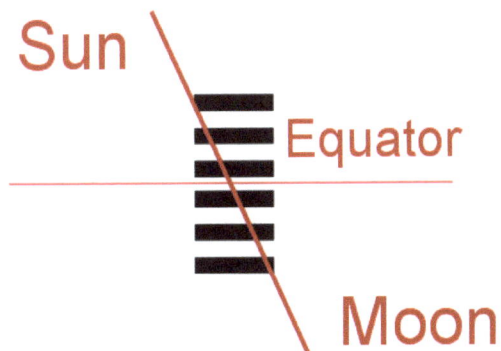

This combination represents the totality of the human experience in time, the full Moon opposite to the Sun, seen from the Earth, to create the basic form of the hexagram.

There are nine cycles in feng shui, combines together they create a larger cycle of one hundred and eighty years. In each of the 19 years period cycle there is a ranging number (a dominating vibration, which is stronger than the others for this period of time) and this vibration is always placed in the center of the grid of the period.

Reigning number	Period
1	1864-1883
2	1884-1903
3	1904-1923
4	5th Feb 1924 - 24th Jan 1944
5	25th Jan 1944 – 12th Feb 1964
6	13th Feb 1964 – 1st Feb 1984

7	2nd Feb 1984 – 21st Jan 2004
8	22nd Jan 2004 – 10th Feb 2024
9	11th Feb 2024 - 2043

All the dates are based on the Chinese Moon calendar (Lunar Year), which is different from the Western calendar. Knowing when the periods start and finish then you can easily calculate the reigning number of the building you live in, so you know what type of energies (vibrations) surround you inside your environment.

To find out the period of a building all you need to know is when the construction of the building is finished.

For example: if you live in a house which was build in 1986, then your house is in period 7 and the grid should look like this:

SE	S	SW
6	2	4

E	5	7	9	W
	1	3	8	
NE		N		NW

After you find the reigning number of the period of the building, remember the rule how to place the rest of the numbers in the square grid.

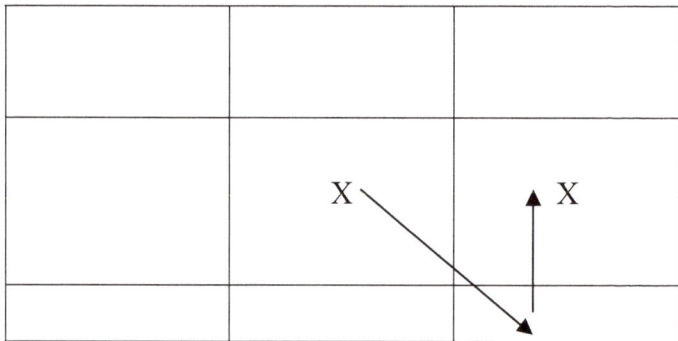

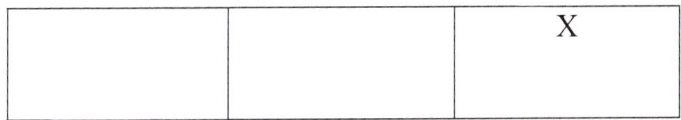

Image 1

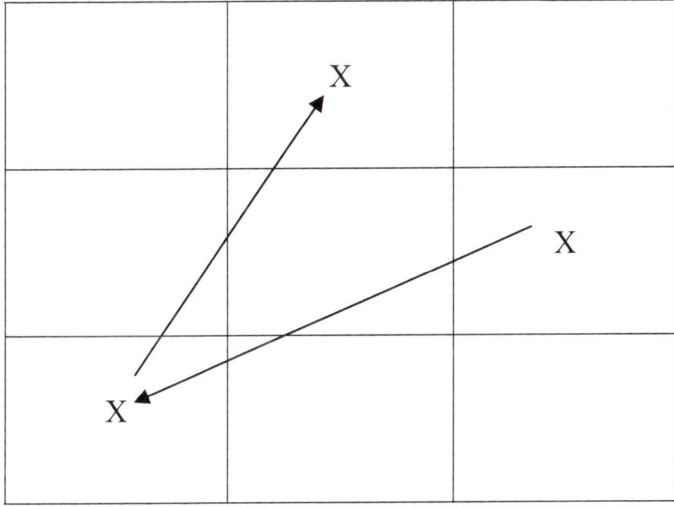

Image 2

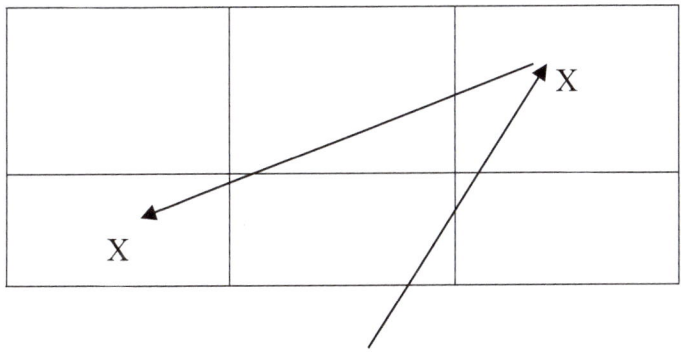

	X	

Image 3

12. Facing direction of a building

The difference in the vibrations of the buildings and their vibrations comes from two more energies places inside. The first one is called water star and it is determent from the facing direction of the building. Let me teach you how to determent the facing direction of a building.

Remember: A facing direction is the direction most open to sunlight. Note that this could be a direction different from the front door. Remember that you have to determent the facing direction of the whole building. People who live in an apartment often get confused and use their front door as a facing direction, which is wrong. If the building is equally open to sunlight then you should look where the road leading to the building is placed.

I will give you ready to use charts for each one of the periods so you don't have to calculate, but you can use them directly into your feng shui analysis.

13. The 9 Periods

Period 1

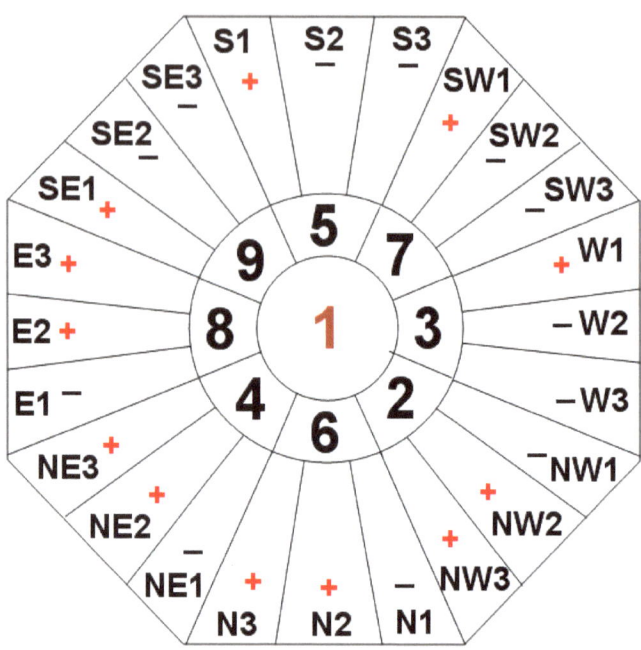

Period 2

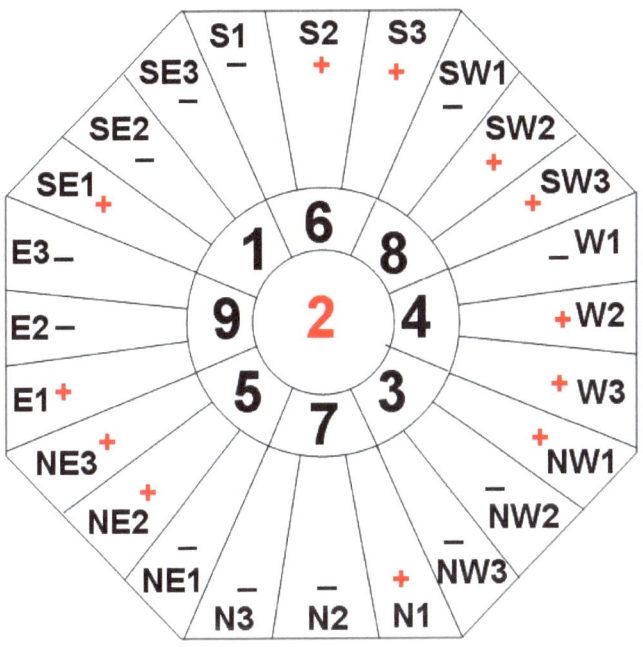

Period 3

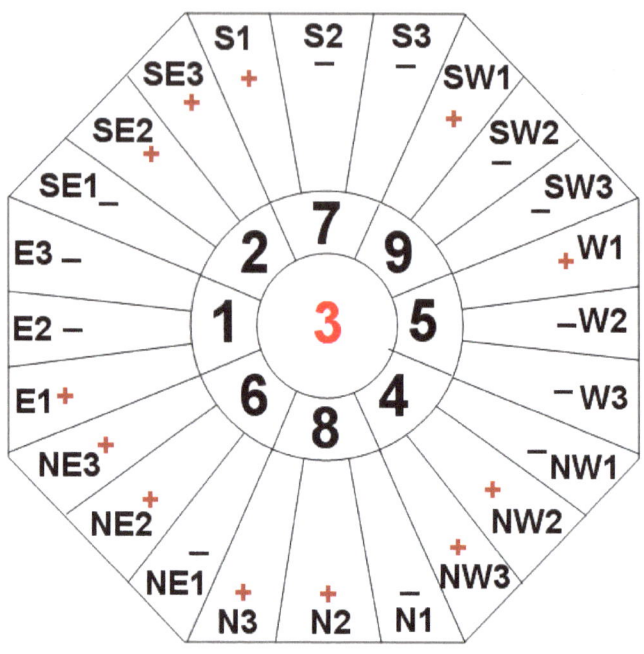

Period 4

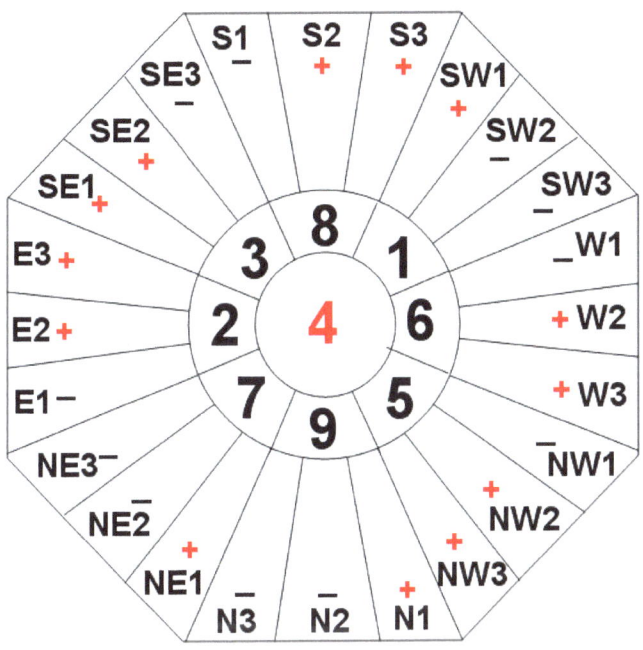

Period 5 also called Lo Shu Square

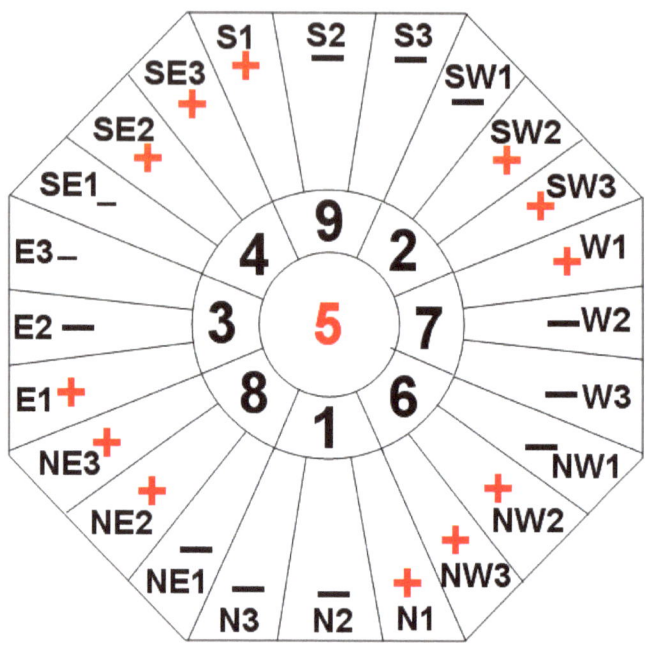

Period 6

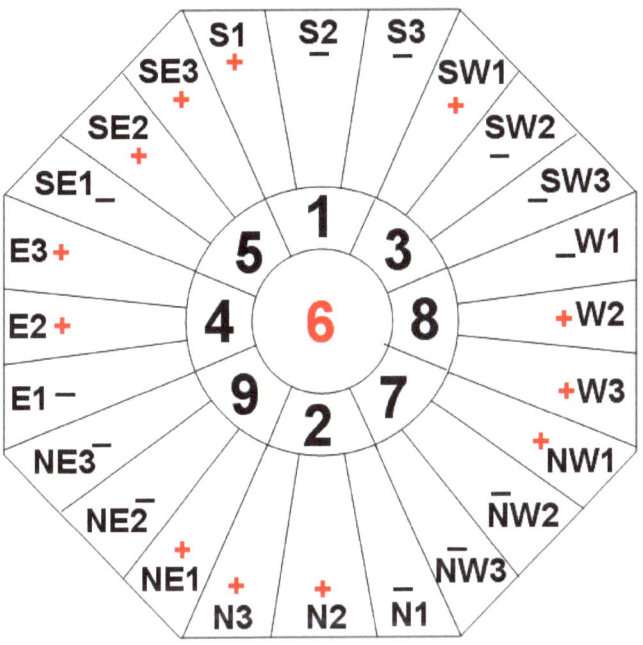

Period 7

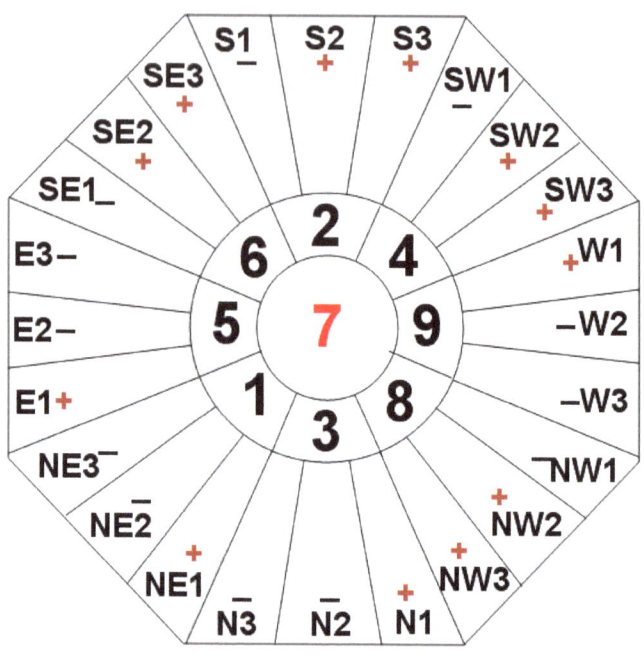

Period 8

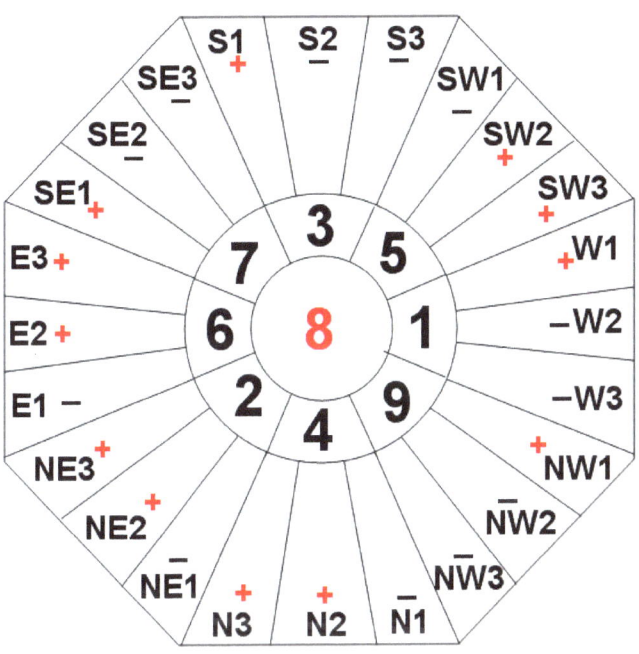

Period 9

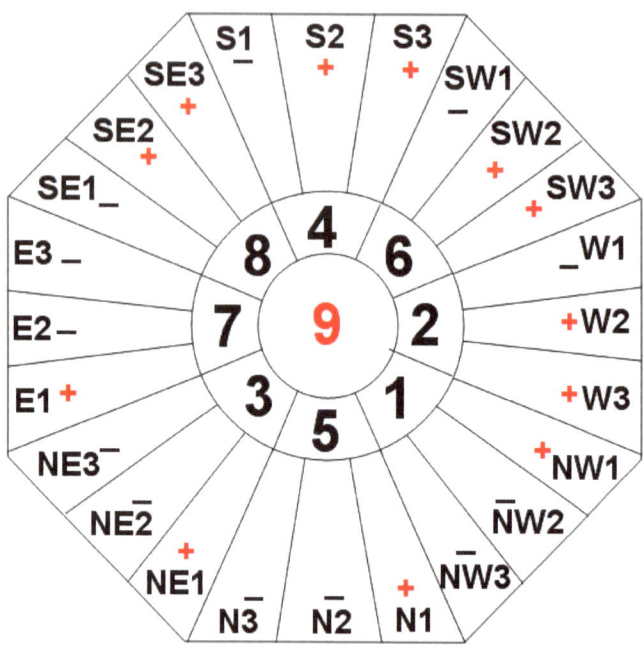

Let us look again an example if the facing direction of the building is 223 degrees of the compass, then its bearing is SW2. Also you should know that the building is in period 8. Then the trigram opposite to the facing star, placed on the back of the building, is called Mountain (Sitting) Star, in our case NE2.

Also have you noticed that each of these facing and sitting stars has a sign + or -? The + and the – indicate the facing star and the mountain star and how they fly in the grid. If the sign flies -++ the star flies in ascending progression. If the signs go +--, then the star flies in descending progression. For instance in our example if the period of the building is 8 and the facing direction is SW2 then if you look at the chart you should see that SW flies-++, then the facing star will fly in ascending progression 5,6,7...etc.

The sitting star NE2 is the trigram 2 and flies -++ also. The chart should look like this:

SE		S		SW
	1 4	6 9	8 2	
	7	3	5	
E	9 3	+2 +5	4 7	W
	6	8	1	
	5 8	7 1	3 6	
	2	4	9	
NE		N		NW

Now you have to learn how to spread these vibrations onto your floor plan. Remember as a rule the natal chart should be spread onto the whole building and if you live in an apartment take a look in which sector or sectors your apartment lays in. If you live in a house, then you should spread the natal chart on the whole floor plan.

The last thing for you to analyze is to see how the trigrams interact between each other in each and every sector so you know whether to activate or exhaust them.

14. The rule of the coherence

Remember this very important rule: In the Universe or in the physics if you want to activate a vibration (a trigram) you should use the same trigram, so you create a coherent pattern. If you want to exhaust a trigram you should use its opposite.

For example if you want to activate the trigram Chien ▬▬ use the same Chien ▬▬trigram (white color). If you want to exhaust the trigram Kun ▬ ▬ (color yllow) use its opposite the Chien ▬▬ trigram (color white). It is that easy.

15. The combinations of the trigrams

Here is a table of the different possible combinations and their meanings:

The combination of trigrams	The result
1 and 1	Excellent for study or research
1 and 2	Marriage problems, danger of miscarriage
1 and 3	Lawsuits and legal problems
1 and 4	Political and media luck, especially for writers.
1 and 5	Health problems
1 and 6	Career luck and promotions, good money luck
1 and 7	Competition
1 and 8	Wealth, misunderstandings between couples or business partners
1 and 9	Excellent career and money

The combination of trigrams	The result
2 and 1	Marriage problems, danger of miscarriage
2 and 2	Illness and accidents
2 and 3	Arguments, legal disputes
2 and 4	Women in the household fight
2 and 5	Total loss, illness
2 and 6	Very good life, power, authority
2 and 7	Problems in conceiving children
2 and 8	Wealth, minor illness
2 and 9	Bad for children, bad luck
3 and 1	Lawsuits
3 and 2	Arguments, legal disputes
3 and 3	Robbery and gossips

The combination of trigrams	The result
3 and 4	Relationship problems
3 and 5	Loss of wealth and money
3 and 6	Limb injuries
3 and 7	Robbery and injuries
3 and 8	Limb injuries for children
3 and 9	Robbery, lawsuits
4 and 1	Political and media luck, especially for writers.
4 and 2	Women in the household fight
4 and 3	Relationship problems with the partner
4 and 4	Romantic relationship
4 and 5	Illness
4 and 6	Good for money, difficulties during pregnancy

The combination of trigrams	The result
4 and 7	Love relationship will suffer, illness of the abdomen
4 and 8	Good for writers, possible limb injury
4 and 9	Academic success, danger of fire
5 and 1	Health problems
5 and 2	Total loss, illness
5 and 3	Loss of wealth and money
5 and 4	Illness
5 and 5	Bad illness
5 and 6	Head illness, bad financial luck
5 and 7	Arguments, illness
5 and 8	Illness to the joints, bones and limbs

The combination of trigrams	The result
5 and 9	Eye problems, danger of fire
6 and 1	Career luck and promotions
6 and 2	Very good life, power, authority
6 and 3	Limb injuries
6 and 4	Good for money, difficulties during pregnancy
6 and 5	Head illness, bad financial luck
6 and 6	Excellent for money and good fortune
6 and 7	Competition over money
6 and 8	Wealth, popularity and great prosperity
6 and 9	Good for money, problems between generations

The	The result

combination of trigrams	
7 and 1	Competition
7 and 2	Problems in conceiving children
7 and 3	Robbery and injuries
7 and 4	Love relationship will suffer, illness of the abdomen
7 and 5	Arguments, illness
7 and 6	Competition over money
7 and 7	Victory over competition
7 and 8	Victory over competition
7 and 9	Danger of fire. Cheating
8 and 1	Prosperity and good luck. Career luck
8 and 2	Wealth. Danger of sickness
8 and 3	Limb injuries
8 and 4	Overpowering mother create problems

The	The result

combination of trigrams	
8 and 5	Illness to the joints, bones and limbs
8 and 6	Wealth, popularity and great prosperity
8 and 7	Victory over competition
8 and 8	Wealth and good luck
8 and 9	Problem between generations.
9 and 1	Excellent career and money
9 and 2	Bad for children, bad luck
9 and 3	Robbery, lawsuits
9 and 4	Academic success, danger of fire
9 and 5	Eye problems, danger of fire
9 and 6	Good for money but there is problems between generations
9 and 7	Danger of fire. Cheating
9 and 8	Problem between generations. Good money fortune.
9 and 9	Danger of fire

There are some special combinations of numbers depending on the direction they are placed. They are called Ho Tu numbers. If you notice them in your chart take advantage of the situation.

Numbers	Benevolent Direction	Malevolent Direction
1 and 6	North: Education luck	South: Accident to the patriarch
2 and 7	South: Financial luck	West: Fatal illness and accidents
3 and 8	East: Success in politics	SW: death by suicide
4 and 9	West: Successful business	East: Children become orphans

At last we come to the so well kept in secret Water Dragon Formula, which brings wealth and money for the household. If you learn how to apply this formula you will have considerable success with money. The formula is based on the Early and Later Heaven Arrangements and their movement, therefore the angle of the water flow and the entrance and exit direction of the water in your property would have a significant importance in the money flow in your life.

16. The Water Dragon Formula

For example: North in Later Heaven Arrangement has the trigram 1, which moves from West in Early Heaven Arrangement to North in Later Heaven Arrangement.

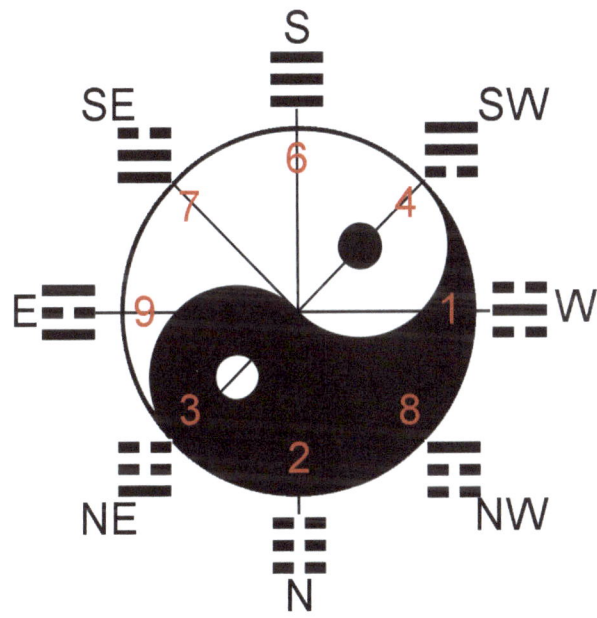

Early Heaven Arrangement

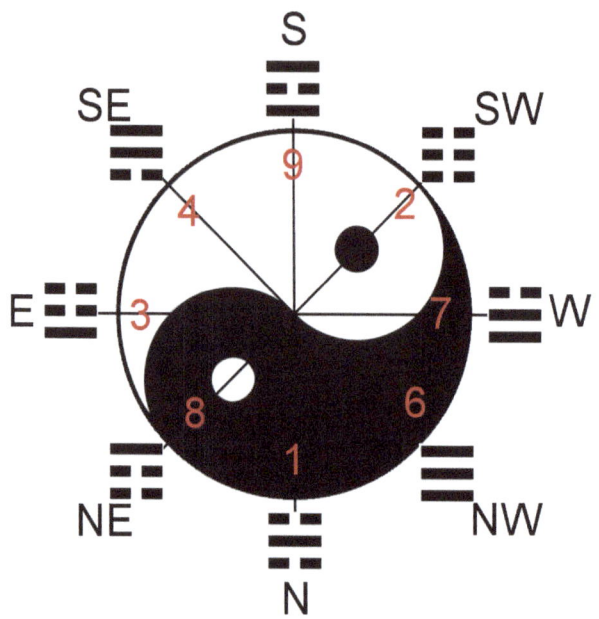

Later Heaven Arrangement

This means that if the water comes from West and goes out to North this will bring an enormous amount of money for the household.

I have created a table for you which can guide you and assist you in the calculation of the Water Dragon Formula for your household.

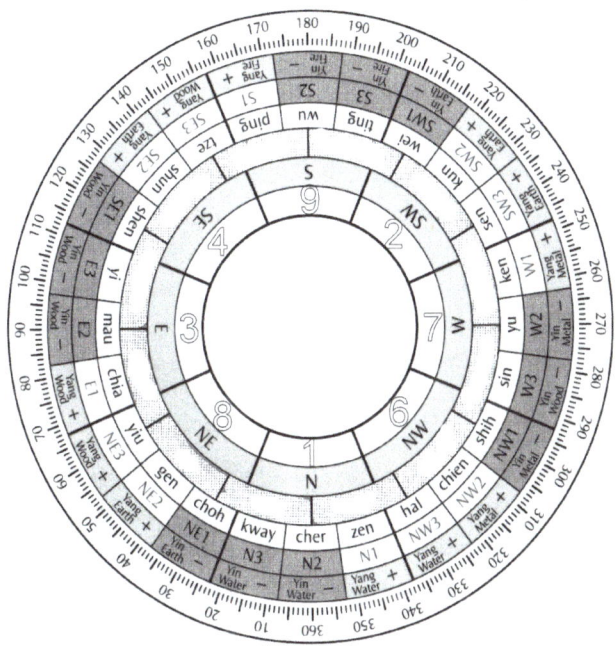

The facing direction of the house is Ping S1 or Wu S2. The water should pass the facing direction and flow out in Sin W3 or Shih NW1 direction between 277.5 and 307.5 degrees from North of the compass. This water flow will bring great success for the household.

The facing direction of the house is Ting S3 or Wei SW1. The water should pass the facing direction and flow out in Zen N1 direction between 337.5 and 352.5 degrees from North.

The facing direction of the house is Kun SW2 or Sen SW3. The water should pass the facing direction and flow out in Yi E3 or Shen SE1 direction between 97.5 and 127.5 degrees from North. This water flow will bring very good fortune especially in business and prosperity for the generations to follow.

The facing direction of the house is Ken W1 or Yu W2. The water should pass the facing direction and flow out in Kway N3 or Choh NE1 direction between 7.5 and 37.5 degrees from North. This will bring long lasting business especially for males.

The facing direction of the house is Sin W3 or Shih NW1. The water should pass the facing direction and flow out in Kun SW2 or Sen SW3 direction between 217.5 and 247.5 degrees from North.

The facing direction of the house is Chain NW2 or Hal NW3. The water should pass the facing direction and flow out in Zen N1 or Cher N2 direction between 352.5 and 7.5 degrees from North. The business will expand enormously.

The facing direction of the house is Zen N1 or Cher N2. The water should pass the facing direction and flow out in Ken direction W1 between 247.5 and 62.5 degrees from North. This direction spells great wealth.

The facing direction of the house is KwayN3 or Choh NE1. The water should pass the facing direction and flow out in Gen NE2 or Yiu direction between 37.5 and 67.5 degrees from North. The family wealth will expand with each child and generation.

The facing direction of the house is Gen NE2 or Yiu NE3. The water should pass the facing direction and flow out in Yi or Shen direction between 97.5 and 127.5 degrees from North. Wealth will grow each year.

The facing direction of the house is Yi E3 or Shen SE1. The water should pass the facing direction and flow out in Gen or Yin direction between 37.5 and 67.5 degrees from North. This direction will bring luxurious life and will be very beneficial for the women in the family.

The facing direction of the house is Shun SE2 or Tze SE3. The water should pass the facing direction and flow out in Kway or Choh direction between 7.5 and 37.5 degrees from North. This direction will bring easy success to the women of the household.

17. The formula of the auspicious directions

The last formula you should know is how to make all these things work for you by calculating your personal auspicious and inauspicious direction. This formula is based on the date of birth based on the lunar calendar.

For example: Let's say the person was born in 1972. Add the last two digits

For a male born before 2000	For a male born after 2000	For a female born before 2000	For a female born after 2000
7+2=9 Deduct the result from 10 10-9=1	7+2=9 Deduct the result from 9 9-1=8	7+2=9 Add the result to 5 9+5=14=1+4=5 *	7+2=9 Add the result to 6 9+6=15=1+5=6
1= ☷	8= ☶	5=8 ☴	6= ☰

*Males with a personal number 5 change to 2, because 5 does not have a trigram. Females with a personal number 5 change to 8 for the same reason.

After you calculate your personal trigram number you can find the auspicious and inauspicious directions from the table below. To make them work for you, you have to face these directions.

People are separated into two groups –east and west group.

 East group are people whose good directions are E, S, N, SE.

West group are people whose good directions are W, NW, NE, SW.

Trigram No	Wealth	Health	Love	Growth	Bad luck	Ghosts	Killing	Total loss	Group
1	SE	E	S	N	W	NE	NW	SE	east
2	N	W	N	S	E	SE	S	N	west

	E		W	W					st
3	S	N	S	E	S	N	N	W	ea
			E			W	W	E	st
4	N	S	E	SE	N	SW	W	N	ea
								E	st
5	Becomes 2 for males and 8 for females								
6	W	N	S	N	S	E	N	S	we
		E	W	W	E				st
7	N	S	N	W	N	S	SE	E	we
	W	W	E						st
8	S	N	W	NE	S	N	E	S	we
	W	W						E	st
9	E	SE	N	S	N	W	S	N	ea
					E		W	W	st

That is all you ever need to know to live a happy, healthy, harmonious and wealthy life.

Good luck to you and thank you for reading my book!

www.ingramcontent.com/pod-product-compliance
Lightning Source LLC
Chambersburg PA
CBHW040310010626

45792CB00022B/68